How to Lose Weight on a Fast Food Diet

V.L. Jenkins

Copyright © 2018 V.L. Jenkins

All rights reserved. No part of this book may be reproduced or transmitted in any form or by any means, electronic or mechanical, including photocopying, recording or by any information storage and retrieval system, without permission in writing from the publisher.

Universal Unlimited Publishing--Detroit, MI
ISBN: 978-0-9996943-0-5
Author: Jenkins, V.L
Title: How to Lose Weight on a Fast Food Diet |
Available Formats: eBook
Paperback distribution

Dedication

Dedicated to my Aunt Mattie Posey, for believing when no one else did.

Chapter One

Do you guys love fast food? If the answer is yes and you're starting to feel guilty don't, because you're not alone. About 80% of Americans eat fast food at least once a week. Have you ever wondered to yourself how can I lose any of this weight if I'm always on the go or just don't have the time in the morning to pack a healthy lunch every day, eat right, exercise and the list goes on. So you end up going to the vending machine and like millions of hard working Americans you hit the drive thru for lunch and sometimes breakfast or dinner. Well here it is the answer to all your weight loss prayers.

I've lived on the road for six years as a truck driver going cross country on a regular basis. Talk about always being on the go. When I first hit the road I had everything planned out including my diet, which including plenty of fruits and vegetables mainly at truck stop salad bars, but as habits go I quickly slid back into being a fast food junkie.

The obvious health risk are always there, greasy foods, high calories, clogged arteries, severe health risk like heart disease and obesity to name a few. Of course all of those facts remain, but it taste so damn good. I mean why else would billions and billions have been and continue to be served. Losing weight is a serious issue especially in America where two-thirds of her citizens are overweight. I'm sure you like many others have tried just about every program under the sun and yet still...

I'm not going to lie or come with some catchy slogan to fuel your inner health nuts. Truth is no matter what diet program you latch onto the real answer to losing weight is you. No one knows your body as well as you, not even your doctor. You know your motivations, your weaknesses, your temptations... speaking of which, which one is yours?

What I have put together with this book is a guide to slowly making change in our daily lives in particular, remember what we put in is what we get out. Tell me this, when you pull into the drive thru at your favorite fast food restaurant what's the first item you usually order for lunch.

For most Americans it's the all familiar cheeseburger and fries usually in the form of some value meal. Well I've done a little research on the classic combo. A typical meal of the value menu (cheeseburger, fries and soft drink) can take your calorie count well up and over 1000 calories, remember around 500 calories a day for lunch is the goal.

When I first walk into my favorite chain (Wendy's) it's hard not to crave one of their mouthwatering juicy 100% beef hamburgers, mines usually was a double with cheese. Moving on to some of the more healthier items on the menu I changed my portions instead of two sandwiches and fries I got one sandwich, then I gradually made the adjustment to small fries, minus the fries all together or substituting them with something else like a baked potato with very little sour cream.

I'm sure there are miracle people out there who could walk away from their cravings without a second thought, such are a rare breed that probably wouldn't need this book or any other book or program. But the reality is most of us just don't have the patience or will to. I did all the research for you guys, but I'm going to need an honest effort from each and every one of you, remember you determine your will to succeed.

The good news is I'm not asking you to go vegan overnight, I've tried it and the cravings I had for meat were monstrous. A week later and I was stuffing my face with double cheeseburgers and strawberry milkshakes. The point is like most things in life losing weight takes time. Sorry... I know this is not what you want to hear especially this early, but like I said I'm not asking for overnight results. Studies show that for the average woman to lose one pound of weight per week she needs to eat about 1500 calories per day calories. An average man needs around 2000 calories. To lose wait at a quicker more expected pace you need to get your metabolism up and that's by eating and burning calories. Little changes such as walking up the office stairs a few times a day, instead of taking the elevator make a big difference. I'm sure as your day goes by you can come up with some pretty creative ways to be active at work (even if you sit at a desk or behind the wheel of a vehicle.) Things such as hand grips and strap on weights help get your blood circulating and that's what you need. You'd be surprise at the little bit of effort it takes to start your transformation into the you, you want to be.

I'm not going to sugar coat the truth, the real key to losing weight isn't the actual plan itself, but your actual commitment to making the changes necessary to achieve your goals. The process starts as the old cliché says, by taking things one day at a time. Whether it be walking a few more steps a day (the max is 10,000 or more steps a day, but I'll get into that later) or stretching during down time. The point I'm making is that the little steps we take at breaking old eating habits will ultimately determine our rate of success.

First I'm going to run down a list of some of the most popular fast food restaurants in the world and go over some of their health benefits and risk. Then I'm going to go to their healthier menu items and add the benefits of making gradual changes. Finally I'm going to give you a mix and match and the diet plan to make it all work. So get ready to eat your way fit.

The myth: *Starving yourself thin is just that a myth, the body was designed to hold out in times of severe* *hunger like how a camel retains water, we retain our fat reserves which is probably why our metabolisms slow down after a certain age to get us through the long haul.*

Step 1

COMMITMENT

To start things off I want to know a little about you. Where do you see yourself six weeks from now? Hopefully if you said looking better and feeling healthier you've come to the right place. But before you turn the pages let's talk history. How many times have you been here before, all ready to take on a life changing challenge, only to lose enthusiasm finding yourself ready to hit the restart button?

Mainly because the topic or fads of the moment tend to get a little boring after a few weeks of trying to somehow incorporate it into your schedule on a regular basis. It's not that the plan or program was necessarily bad, it's just adding it in wasn't a good fit, so like me you probably abandoned them. I have a bunch of infomercial junk in my basement closet do you? The trick to it is finding something that doesn't conflict with your way of life then slowly adjusting to it until it becomes habit or routine.

The most important thing to any form of success is the desire to stay successful. Now of course we all know that with addition there must also be subtraction. Meaning a lot of things we like are going to either be eliminated or cut back from the menu. Sorry, but you can't have a shake with every meal and still be successful.

Pushing yourself into doing something isn't good either, because you burnout quickly and before you know it you're adding to that collection in the basement closet. The only one who can make those changes is you and losing weight is about getting healthy all around. So basically you have to know you, through and through.

What I'm asking you to do is put your cravings to the side, believe in yourself, and put forth the effort, because just a little commitment can get you over that hump. Don't worry I'm not asking you to eat carrots and celery for dinner, but some of the more heavy helpings that stick to your ribs will have to be lightened up some.

Experimenting is a big step toward making change, it involves a little thing called variety, which is said to be the spice of life.

Trying new things never hurts and finding new delight in choosing healthier foods makes eating less boring and not the race of finding that one particular food fix.

No pain no gain, no risk no reward, no guts no glory, the list of encouraging expressions goes on and all have the same point. If you don't do what you want to be done than it won't be, meaning somewhere in all of us lays a warrior that's ready to take charge. The problem is that acting upon this in the real world requires work and sweat.

And it's not like people don't have the ability to free their self at will, it's just that the hustle and bustle of everyday life (work, family, personal affairs...etc.) get in the way of that freedom. Work is work no matter if you're lifted car engines or pushing keypads, either way you are working. And after a long day relaxing sounds like nirvana. So who has time to exercise and eat right? Believe it or not you do, and I'm going to help you. So ready or not here we go.

BEST PICKS

ARBY's
Although it isn't the typical fast food restaurant, a lot of their menu items haves less calories than most of the others. Eating roast beef over greasy hamburgers is a no-brainer. Items like their Chicken breast Filet, Sourdough Egg & Cheese or Original Roast Beef sandwich offer lower calories making Arby's an ideal restaurant to eat healthy.

BURGER KING
Burger King is known for their flame broiled burgers opposed to the more common cousins in the fast food industry. One item they serve is a Veggie burger. They just don't get any healthier than that, but the taste you're expecting when you bite into that bun is **a** surprise. Eating these over regular hamburgers will definitely put you on the right path, but eating fast food comes down to taste and some people just can't get used to it. Other items they offer like Chili, which is a great choice and the Whopper Jr. minus the bacon or Fire Grilled Salads offer a

reasonable amount of calories.

SUBWAY

In terms of fast food you can't go wrong with Subway, they offer a variety of lean meats and fresh vegetables that can slim you down if you go cold turkey or oven roasted. There are plenty of choices you can make for fresh tasting low calorie meals. Chicken and Turkey sandwiches being the healthiest or a bowl of their delicious soups or chowders. Remember to pack on the veggies and lighten up the sauce for maximum effect.

WENDY'S

Like many other Americans this happens to be my personal favorite. The burgers they serve can be monstrous in size and oh so tasty. Having a burger these days is not something I do often, but Dave sure did know what he was doing. Lots of items on the menu these days lean towards the healthier side such as the Chicken Grill Sandwich, Small Chili and Baked potato to name a few.

KFC

The thought of eating chicken over beef in

regards to weight loss are justified, easier to digest and fewer calories make it the ideal food. Problem is that when we order our chicken on the go it's usually tossed in a batch of grease that adds onto the fat intake making the bird less healthy than the beef. Ordering your food grilled or baked will take that entire extra out of the picture. The majority of the items on their menu however are deep fried, and most people love them for their famous 11 herbs and spices after being thrown in the fat. Another item that can load on the calories is their potatoes wedges, thick cut fries that can be more fattening than the meal. Not many items they offer are on the light side, but switching to grilled chicken will only help. Some of their ideal items would be the sides like corn on the cob, baked beans and mashed potatoes and gravy opposed to potatoes wedges.

MC DONALDS

Is the number one fast food chain in America. So big that they actually have a say so in the way ground beef is produced within the beef industry, being their largest purchaser. Now that's pull! The items on their menu are geared to fatten you up and keep you coming back for more, Supersize any one? Finding something healthy on their menu can be tricky, your best choices would be the Fruit 'n' Yogurt Parfait and McArtesian.

TACO BELL

Tacos are naturally a fattening food, fried ground beef dressed in cheese and loaded with sauce. The calories skyrocket from there and who can eat just one taco. The trick to their menu is ordering your tacos without cheese (Fresco style) and lighten up on the sauce, but sometimes that still might not be enough. Experimenting with items like their Chicken Soft Taco, Chicken enchilada without the cheese and loaded with veggies. The Bean Burrito or burrito Steak Supreme, again minus the cheese is also pretty good choices.

Step 2

MANAGING YOUR METABOLISM

Before we go on let's look into some of our eating habits and the products we eat. Old sayings are still around for a reason, it's because there's some fact to them one way or another. And the one about breakfast being the most

important meal of the day is no different.
First off what is metabolism and what does it do? It's kind of like an energy converter for our body the more we rev it up by eating and staying active, the more fat we burn. Think of food as fuel, when you go to the gas tank and get a fill up you never leave the pump in your gas tank, fuel would be spilling all over the place. The same goes for our bodies, when you overeat food ends up spilling all over the place instead of just in our stomach where it's converted into energy. Like any running machine the body needs a constant supply of energy for even a menial task such as breathing.

The name of the game is burning calories and keeping your metabolism revved up. Some people think that if I starve myself then pig out I won't gain weight because I made room for extra. Truth is that when you hold off on eating to eat more lately, your metabolism slows down and has to pick back up. So that large second helping you had tends to burn slower than if you had ate just enough at interval times of the day.

Not eating is also not healthy, when you starve yourself to lose weight your body begins getting the energy it needs by taking away from muscle, which leads to unhealthy weight loss. Remember you have to keep your metabolism active to lose weight, which means you have to eat consistently, not overeat but enough to keep it running (which means until you're full and you don't feel hungry anymore). Some people confuse hunger with thirst so I recommend drinking water more.

Being active, such as playing sports or hitting the gym rev your metabolism into overdrive. But remember the *food as fuel rule* the more you put in your tank the more active you'll need to be.

Also remember it all starts with attitude, staying positive will increase your chances of success. Stress plays a part in weight gain. Try listening to meditative music during lunch or one of your breaks, anything that relaxes you. The key is to find time to take your mind off your concerns at some point during your day. Stay positive. Just like your body your brain needs rest as well, before it overloads from work, the kids, stress or life in general.

Even though you don't have much time for

lunch, be sure to let your food digest and settle in your stomach properly. Think of your stomach as a food disposal, the more you clog in there at once the more possibility something may get stuck. Please don't take that the wrong way. What I'm saying is that like anything else your stomach needs time to get ready for what's coming next.

Yes our metabolism does slow as we get older, but staying active during the day at work helps keep your metabolism running and eventually helps you burn calories. The trick to losing weight goes back to elementary, doing the math. This means to lose weight all you have to do is eat less calories and burn more. Around 500 calories a day for lunch would be the goal, but with a life constantly on the go who has time to stop and do the math? Overall if you stay active you will lose weight with this method. A job that keeps you moving really helps the blood circulate which gets those muscles that aid in fat burning into the game.

But what if you spend your day behind a desk or the wheel of a vehicle, what happens to your metabolism then? Well of course the opposite so how do you keep it moving? I'll let you know a little later in Step 4.

DIGESTION

Your digestive health has a lot to do with weight loss. Feeling bloated, gassy, or just irregular can affect the plans you made by interfering with your metabolism. Your stomach produces a chemical hormone when you get hungry that tells your brain it's time to eat. When we overeat we cause a chemical imbalance that can send mixed signals to your brain making you feel hungry all the time.

Large helpings of sugar or in most products high fructose corn syrup add to the problem. When we ignore the signs of being full the food for fuel rule is broken and food becomes pleasure. I'm not saying that it's wrong to enjoy our food, that's the reason we have taste buds. No, but eating for the sake of eating can trigger this. Too much overeating can be a sign of food addiction so watch out.

So how do you manage your cravings and lose weight? We start by taking fatty foods out of our diets and find appropriate good tasting and healthier substitutes. Fast food may go down fast but it takes time to process in the stomach. Adjusting your diet can take time especially if you're constantly on the go. The best way to get started is early and by early I mean breakfast. Eating a well-balanced breakfast every morning or so can help your body adjust to the changes. Eating cereals rich in fiber and whole grains are a healthy choice.

Eating fruit and vegetables are a quick way to lose weight, if you can afford to eat this way every day and have the tolerance to eat large helpings every day. I would recommend buying produce from a fruit market. They're much better for your budget. Adding slices of fruit in your cereal up the taste and give you a nutritious breakfast.

Try some alternatives at breakfast such as using honey and ground cinnamon as sweeteners as an exception to sugar. Eating slices of fruit or mixing smoothies can help with metabolism early in the morning and taking some with you to work can stop those routine trips to the pop machine. Switching from coffee to honey sweetened green tea can also increase your metabolism and lower stress levels as well. Eating hot cereal such as Cream of Wheat, as opposed to cold. You'll want to cook it yourself instead of just using instant ready pouches that have already been sweetened.

Water also helps with digestion so be sure to drink plenty of water through the work day as many bottles or trips to the water fountain as you can. Drinking the recommended 8 glasses of water will help flush out your system and get things working properly and help with some of those cravings.

Having digestive problems can be a sign that we're not giving our stomach time to digest what we've been eating. Things should flow smooth, those over the counter drugs that can help with these problems are miracle medicines, but also a sign that we're eating for pleasure. I would recommend getting a juicer and a recipe book, lots of natural foods can help with digestion problems such as diarrhea and indigestion.

Here are a few foods that help stimulate metabolism:

Egg Whites:
Egg whites are rich in branched-chain amino acids, which keep your metabolism going. Eggs are also loaded with protein and vitamin D.

Lean meats:
Lean meats like chicken are full of iron which helps to keep the metabolism from slowing down. Deficiencies in this mineral can slow our metabolism. Eat three to four daily servings of iron-rich foods, such as chicken or turkey.

Chili peppers:
These spicy veggies contain chemicals that can naturally boost your metabolism. They contain vitamin C, Vitamin B-6, Vitamin A, and Capsaicin, a chemical compound that can boost your metabolism into high gear.

Green Tea:
This drink has been popular for centuries and contains a compound that helps in fat burning. The secret to green tea's power is epigallocatechin gallate (EGCG). This potent antioxidant works by reducing the amount of fat your body absorbs, which it helps speed the weight loss process.

Whole grains:
Whole food requires more work to break down, they help in the fat burning process by causing the body to use more to digest. Eating whole foods **like oatmeal** can help increase

thermogenesis, which aids in fat burning and contain a high nutrient density, high in protein, vitamin B, mineral and fiber.

Lentils:
Are dried beans and legumes that come in several varieties. They are a very good source of dietary fiber, copper, phosphorus, and magnesium, which is good for the circulatory system and also aids in the fight against deadly disease. Also lentils provide help in keeping your blood sugar normal, so anyone dealing with diabetes eating more could help you.

Also they are a good source for protein, iron, vitamin B, zinc, potassium. They also contain antioxidants that help prevent certain cancers, such as colon cancer. The fiber they provide keeps your digestive system running smoothly and lower chances for heart disease.

Water:
When we get dehydrated our metabolisms slow down. Drinking water helps tremendously in weight loss forcing you to feel full a lot quicker than normally. Drinking water fills you up so you tend to be less hungry throughout the day. I recommend drinking eight 8-ounce glasses, which equals about 2 liters, or half a gallon a day for maximum effect.

NO FRIES

One of the unhealthiest foods that we eat almost with every fast food combo is fried potatoes or French fries more commonly. In fact you have a better chance of obesity, diabetes and heart disease if you scarf them down on a regular basis than any other food on the menu. Though technically you are eating vegetables, the deep frying in oil takes away from the benefits and add to the health risk.

The calories we get in an order of small fries can be up to 300 plus and when you start super sizing you can double or triple that depending on your restaurant of choice. Usually they are prepped ahead of time in oils to aid in shelf life, before they even get tossed in the deep fryer and hit your tray. The fat in them sticks to you longer simply because you're taking in so much of it at a single time. Studies showed that the average American who ate fast food often usually had up to four helpings per week. The amounts of oil in those fries would almost be like drinking a small cup worth.

Also the salt on there can be as much as 1000mg worth, and if you add on some more, well. Sodium chloride taken in such high amounts can increase the chances of high blood pressure, heart attack and stroke among other things. Cutting back or cutting out the fries from your meal completely will help weight loss. I highly recommend making steps towards this, doing so will leave you feeling less sluggish after you eat. Try replacing them with healthier items of the menu like baked potatoes or side salad.

HIGH FRUCTOSE CORN SYRUP
One of the most popular products in stores and fast food restaurants are soda pop. Just about everyone in the world has had some form of manufactured pop. This is where many Americans get their source of water to keep from being dehydrated. Although the water is clearly there what else is there isn't quite so clear to the public. High Fructose Corn Syrup is one of the most printed words on the ingredients labels for most products in store and just about every bottle or can of pop. There are sodas with natural sources of sweetness like pure sugar, but they tend to be a little more expensive.

When you order that value combo at Mc Donald's with a super-size soft drink you're overloading yourself with a calorie building liquid that over time only adds to weight gain and contributes to failing health. Try switching your favorite soda with a flavored water, with slices of fresh fruit to add some taste.

Unsweetened or lightly sweetened tea will help your weight loss efforts tremendously. Soft drinks are like bad carb thrown in a blender then swallowed down after every bite of the meal we're eating. In other words they add to the problem by speeding up the weight gain. Not drinking soft drinks and eating fast food seem impossible? Let put that to the test. Here are a few substitute items from some of your favorite restaurants. Have a go.

Iced Tea

Low Fat Milk

Water with fruit splashes

So why cut back, well heavy consumption of High Fructose Corn Syrup has been linked to obesity especially in children. Also chances for development of diabetes, which becomes a prolonged health condition increase from overindulgence along with heart disease, liver damage, and hypertension with the possibility of having a stroke as well. Now this is only a warning that excessive use of products that contain it can overtime present signs of these problems.

Avoiding foods and drinks that are sweetened with it can be difficult. Almost every label you find in a modern super market has it printed on it. So going cold turkey is your choice, remember to cut back on your intake to help speed up the weight loss process.

One way to start would be switching to diet sodas. Flavored waters are just as tasty, but be sure to check the label because some do contain HFCS. Sparkling mineral water such as Perrier is a good healthy alternative, adding a splash of fresh fruit (which can be purchased at some your favorite fast food places in the form of a fruit cup) can give it some sweet flavor.

Step 3

HEALTHY SNACKING
There's a reason you start to feel hungry a few hours after you've had breakfast, for me usually somewhere around 10:00 am. During this time I

find myself making my way towards the vending machines a couple hours before my lunch break, sound familiar. These cravings can come like clockwork every few hours, one way to manage this is by eating a snack every so often. You don't have to feel guilty about this either, but changing that Butterfingers for a Granola bar is the price.

When you do decide to hit the vending-machine, a good alternative to those all too familiar candy bars is a bag of nuts like peanuts, cashews or almonds. They're loaded with fiber, unsaturated fats, omega-3 fatty acids, vitamin E and protein. Choose unsalted nuts to help keep down your sodium consumption.

Here are a few healthy selections

Granola Bar
Granola bars are usually made with whole grains remarkably with less than 200 calories a serving making them a tasty healthier choice instead of candy bars.

Popcorn
Plain low-calorie popcorn is a whole grain food that studies have found to contain a small level

of antioxidants, believed to aid in disease-fighting. Although not the healthiest alternative, especially when you eat the flavored types that add high amounts of sugar and calories from butter.

Sunflower Kernels
Sunflower seeds offer various nutritional benefits like vitamin E, copper, vitamin B, phosphorus, thiamine, and **selenium**. Also remember to try for the unsalted variety.

Fig Newton's
Fig Newton's are a better choice than cookies and candy bars. One reason they actually are made with real fruit and with whole grains. Figs are heavy in fiber **magnesium**, manganese, **calcium** (which promotes bone density), copper, and **potassium** (which helps lower blood pressure), as well as vitamins, principally K and B6.

Pretzels
A bag of plain unflavored pretzel can be a good alternative snack, loaded with iron, zinc and **folate**. And besides these nutrients, pretzels are low in fat. Hold up, though, this snack can come at the price of too much salt, because some brands of pretzels have nearly a day's supply of **sodium** in one serving.

Yogurt
This tasty dairy snack offer health benefits like calcium, potassium, vitamin B, magnesium. It also helps out your digestive system with gastrointestinal conditions like diarrhea when regularly incorporated into your diet.

Step 4

STAYING ACTIVE

WALK IT OFF
Exercise and weight lose go together like not exercising and gaining weight. You have to get your muscles active to burn fat and your heart pumping to supply the blood needed to these areas. Sitting at a desk for seven or more hours makes achieving this a little bit more difficult. Time management comes into play and a few minutes a day of walking extra steps can turn into shed calories and eventually pounds. Our metabolisms run faster when we exercise and walking though it may seem tedious qualifies. Using a pedometer helps to monitor your progress and makes it less of a guessing game.
The goal would be between 6000 and 12,000 steps a day. This takes time and some of us just

don't have it to spare. So what do you do? You can start by taking the stairs at work each and every day. Avoiding the elevator and walking across the parking lot instead of parking close to the entrance whether at work or shopping. Treadmills count as well so investing in one may be a good idea. If possible to obtain one with an incline do so to get the maximum effect out of your workout. Remember to add an upbeat soundtrack of some of your favorite tunes to the mix to take away any boredom you may encounter.

EXERCISE
When we stay active we speed up the heart, which gets the blood pumping and boost up our metabolism which raises our energy levels. All of these are essential for a lasting effect of weight loss. Strength training such as walking with ankle or wrist weights helps keep the muscles primed to aid in burning up calories. If you ate a more balanced healthy diet every day and walked at least 10-12,000 steps a day using strap on weights, you will see the results sooner than later. Going to the gym is a plus, but will have little effect without changes in our eating habits. Riding a bike to work if you can afford the time

is a quick way to keep active especially if you're sitting behind a desk all day.

OFFICE YOGA

When you sit behind a desk for eight or more hours a day five days out of the week your chances at losing weight decrease. One reason is your circulatory system including your heart requires you to be active to aid in the process.

When your legs go to sleep and get really numb, that's a sign of circulation being temporarily cut. So how do you find a solution, who has time to stop at the gym every night? Walking the halls and steps instead of taking the elevator is a start.

Another would be to take advantage of down time by stretching your arms and legs right from your chair. I know what it sounds like, but there are some stress relieving poses that will get your blood flowing and not freak out your coworkers.

Here are a few to try out at work

1. Seat Back
Just take in a large breath
While reaching for the sky with your arms spread wide.
Now bend your upper body back keeping
Your spine straight, hold breath, release and repeat.

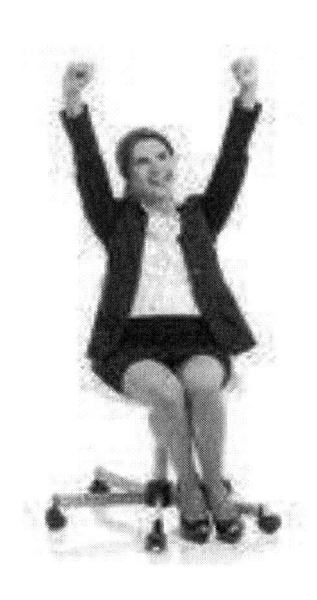

2. Seat Twist

Sit straight take in a breath, rotate Your side using your core muscles holding armrest release, switch sides and repeat. Staying straight is important and Tightening your core muscles.

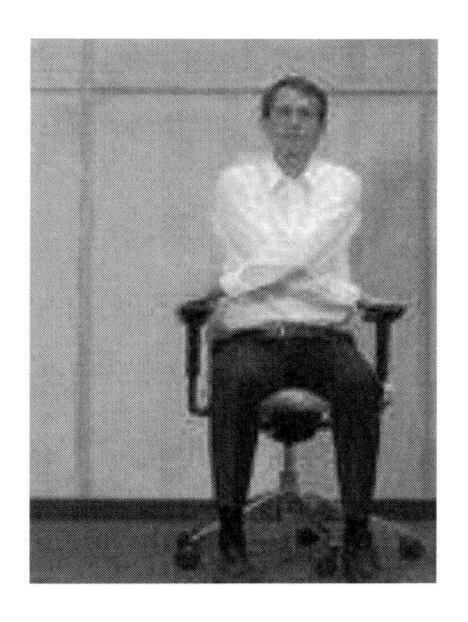

3. Wrist Bend extend arm in front of you,
Bend elbow slightly then bend wrist in
All directions separately.
Next bend fingers inward towards wrist
As far as comfortable.
Release and shake arms to stimulate circulation.
This should really help keyboard cramp.

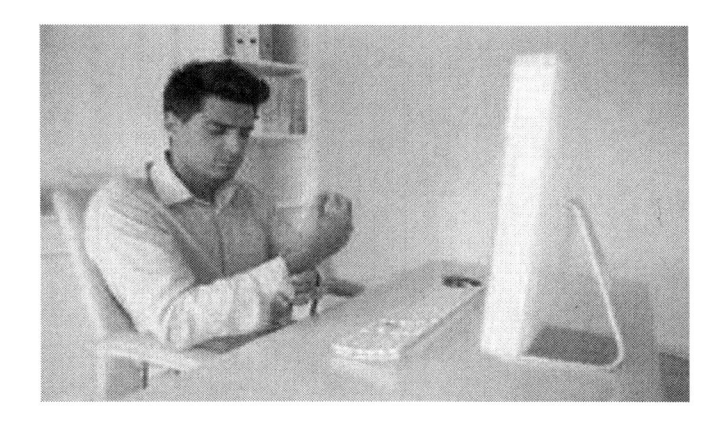

4. Desk Stretch Pull chair away desk

Step about arm's length away then drop head Between shoulders extending arms on to the desk. Your spine should be straight to help any hunching back feeling you may have from inactivity and leaning over your keyboard all day at work.

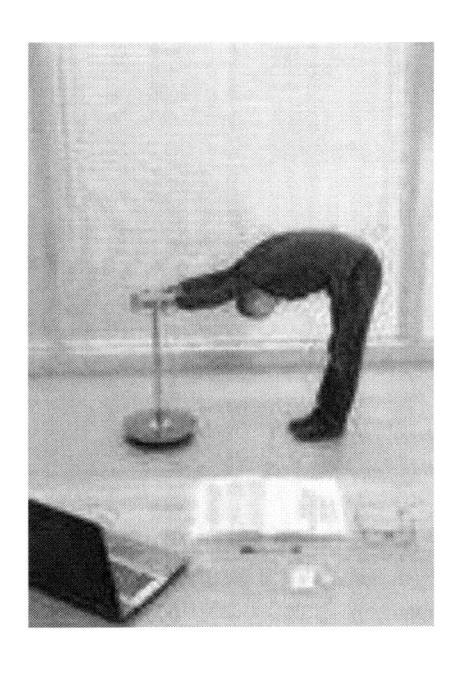

5. Forward Stretch

Okay let's get out of the chair.
Standing on the side of your desk reach over
As low as possibly comfortable.
Hold position for 20 breaths. Release and repeat.
Be sure to keep loose to allow better circulation.

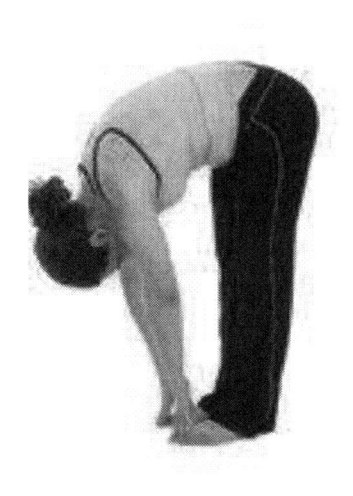

6. Lotus

Sit back with your neck slightly elevated,
Raise your arms open palmed with index finger locked to thumb.

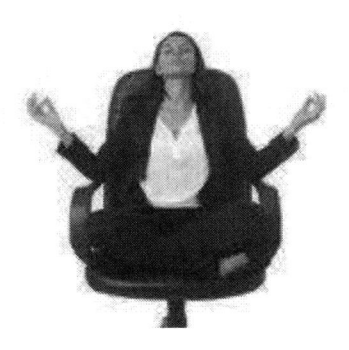

This can be used to relax the mind and body. Folding the legs if at all possible to relieve your spine.

7. Restoration With arms folded in front of you across on your desk, rest your head face down and allow time between positions for your body to adjust, especially if you've pushed yourself.

Step 5

MAKING HEALTHY LIFESTYLE CHANGES
Okay before we go any further we're going to have to make some changes in some of those habits that add to the problem. Losing weight and remaining healthy come from adjusting you dour eating habits and the way we take care of our physical health. Hopefully this guide can help with some of those changes. Like I said nobody knows you like you do so take your time and find the right alternatives to benefit your lifestyle.

BREAKFAST
When we eat a healthy breakfast it provides us with the energy we need to get our day going. Eating breakfast prevents early morning hungriness, reducing the number of snacks (if any) that we have before lunch time. Skipping breakfast could leave you feeling sluggish and lacking concentration. So make time to eat a

nutritious breakfast it provides energy for the activities during the morning and helps to prevent that mid-morning slump.

Here a few healthy items you should add to your breakfast menu. You can prepare them in 10 minutes or less.

Bagel with low fat cream cheese.
Vegetable omelet.
Oatmeal with fresh fruit slices.
Scrambled eggs.
Whole grain, granola bars, breakfast bars.
Yogurt.
French toast.
Egg whites.
Whole grain cereals, with fresh fruit (bananas, blueberries, raspberries, strawberries, or nuts).

JUICING

When you wake up in the morning with a tall glass of freshly squeezed fruit or vegetables juice not only do you get all the nutrients your body needs to get going for the day such as an wonderful abundance of vitamins, potassium, calcium, but you feel energized and full of life, it's almost a natural high. And since you're filling up with a tall glass you shouldn't feel hungry until lunch or an early morning snack.

The combinations you can make with a juice machine are endless and throwing things like ginger root gives it a powerful kick of disease fighting power. Your risk of serious diseases like cancer and heart disease are dramatically reduced if you juice every day.

SMOOTHIES

Early in the morning when the chaos of the day is just beginning you need a breakfast that's going to be both tasty and nutritious. With such a short amount of time to prepare for the work day (depending on when you normally get up, I usually give myself an hour to get ready) you really can miss the most important meal of the day. These filling treats can only speed up the process by lowering your early morning calories intake leaving room for lunch. Popping some fresh fruit and veggies in the blender can solve this dilemma. Naturally sweet and lower in calories than most sweet treats, smoothies satisfy hunger and help start your day of right.

Buying your smoothies from across the counter can never be as safe as making your own. Remember they want you to keep coming back for more so they may pour in the sugar just to sweeten the deal. The alternative making them yourself means you know exactly what you're getting. I wrote down a few quick recipes that will leave you feeling energized and ready for your day check them out and enjoy.

Try using soy, almond or skim milk.

Cram-Raspberry
2 cups of frozen raspberry
1 ½ cups of cranberries
½ small
2 cubes of ice

Blend all ingredients until creamy.
Add ice until smooth.
Pour in glass

Green detox
1 ½ cups of parsley
2 peeled cucumber
2 apples
2 cups of spinach
1 cup cut celery

Blend all ingredients until creamy.

Add ice until smooth.
Pour in glass

Banana Strawberry
2 peeled bananas
1 cup fresh strawberry
1 cup sweetened almond milk
1 small low fat strawberry yogurt

Blend all ingredients until creamy.
Add ice until smooth.
Pour in glass

Pineapple Prize
1 sliced pineapple
1 mango (pitted)
½ inch of ginger root
1cup of coconut water

Blend all ingredients until creamy.
Add ice until smooth.
Pour in glass

Grapefruit Citrus
2 grapefruits
1 orange
½ honeydew melon

2 kiwi
¼ cup of natural yogurt
Blend all ingredients until creamy.
Add ice until smooth.
Pour in glass

Kiwi Lime
2 peeled kiwi
2 apples
½ lime peeled
2 ice cubes

Blend all ingredients until creamy.
Add ice until smooth.
Pour in glass

Blueberry Blast
2 cup of frozen or fresh blueberries
1 small low fat blueberry yogurt
½ cup of frozen or fresh blackberries
½ cup frozen or fresh raspberries

Blend all ingredients until creamy.
Add ice until smooth.
Pour in glass

Cherry Champagne
2 cups of pitted cherries
½ cup of cranberries
1 inch ginger root
1 cup of sparkling mineral water

Blend all ingredients until creamy.
Add ice until smooth.
Pour in glass

Waterberry
1 cup of frozen or fresh strawberries
2 cups of sliced watermelon
¼ sliced beet
½ honeydew melon

Blend all ingredients until creamy.
Add ice until smooth.
Pour in glass

Carrot Orange
2 carrots
3 oranges
1 apple
1 inch ginger root

Blend all ingredients until creamy.

Add ice until smooth.
Pour in glass

ALCOHOL

Alcoholic beverages such as beer, wine or mixed drinks should be kept to a minimal. Not only to prevent substance abuse, which causes 80 plus thousand deaths a year, but because it's full of calories that can put the weight you worked so hard to keep off right back on you. The saying is that a glass of wine may be good for the heart, but three or four is bad for weight loss.

SOFT DRINKS

Carbonated drinks like pop and sweetened juices are the main ingredients in the calorie account of most Americans. It's like pouring sugar down your mouth and washing it down with water and artificial flavors. One of the **main** causes of diabetes, we averagely consume at least an average of 44.7 gallons per person, per year. The High Fructose only adds to weight gain and it's in just about in everything we drink.

Lots of organic products like 100% all natural juices are available and serve as a good replacement to those convenient 2 liters we're so use to buying, but drinking too much can be bad due to high calorie and sugar counts. Drinking flavored water with your meal is a kickoff to not drinking soft drinks, at least not so much. Cutting them out all together will tremendously increase your chances at success. Try drinking green tea or naturally flavoring your water yourself by adding fruit.

FRIES
Simply put if you eat fries with every meal especially medium or large, than losing weight is out of the question. The calories in the fries alone will double on top of your meal. Also overeating fries has been proven to cause disease like cancer or heart attack. Truth is like most people I liked to have fries and a burger, but the facts still remain so making lifestyle changing choices is up to you. And the salt on them can only add to the risk. Eating a baked potato can be an easy way to transition from fries or baking them in the oven.

FOOD ADDICTION
Sugar is substituted in our foods through ingredients like HFCS, saccharin, sucralose, aspartame, the list goes on. These artificial

sweeteners can cause craving for more sugar throughout the day in foods like chocolate, which itself can bring on addiction.

Cheese also can get you addicted, who orders a hamburger over a cheeseburger? The fat content in it however will keep the pounds on and coming. Low fat cheese can help if you cook with it or eat it on a regular basis.

When we eat without being hungry it comes from a chemical imbalance that triggers cravings similar to drug addiction. Now I'm not saying that the two can be compared, but the similarities are there. So what to do when you got a taste for a big bowl of ice cream? Have it, but don't overdo it with another and another. Addiction is powerful and sometimes sheer willpower won't do. Giving in is not something to feel guilty about, things take time. So if you sneak off and have a slice of hot apple pie with ice cream forgive yourself. Remember how you felt after and try not to repeat it and reawaken your guilty conscience.

The key here is not cutting foods you love out, but changing your eating habits around them.

Being addicted to food can also come from other things like being depressed, upset or bored. Some people can't even watch TV without having something to eat. Incorporating exercise in your routine will cut back these cravings especially if you drink plenty of water after.

The strongest thing to breaking this addiction will be family support, when you have to sneak off to eat those unmentionable snacks they become less attractive. Running down to the store for a candy bar isn't as appealing as reaching in the fridge for one.

Change your refrigerator by stocking up on healthier snacks and foods. The foods we eat because of taste alone should be traded for similar tasting products with less harmful ingredients. Replacing ice cream and candy bars with yogurt and granola bars helps.

Not dining in can be a big help in your weight loss plans. When we sit down and eat the temptations to go back for seconds or thirds only increase and we tend to eat more food and spend more money. Fortunately or unfortunately depending on how you look at it, most of us on our lunch breaks don't have time to sit there and eat.

DINNER:
The last meal of the day normally is the biggest and when you add on the seconds it can become overbearing. Right before you call it a night you should be gearing your body up to go to work while you get some well-deserved rest. Our metabolism slows down a bit when we sleep and packing on the extra calories only leads to packing on the pounds. The facts are clear though to some they may seem harsh, but eating the way you did before you decided to make your changes just won't work.

Number 1, you really have to ask yourself how serious you are about making the change to the new you. Because it takes change to make change and eating those fried greasy foods we grew up on is going to have to at some point come to an end.

Eating a variety of vegetables is more than enough to promote healthy weight loss. The thing is though that there's not much taste to eating them raw, which is the most effective way to gain their health inducing benefits.

Stir frying or sautéing them can add flavor without destroying all the nutritional value. Adding them to the dinner table every night will help fill you up with less fattening food before you go to bed, when our metabolism slows down.

Eating at a buffet is a treat for the whole family with foods from every corner of the map being offered. It's pretty hard to visit one and not find some of your personal favorites available. Some people like to wait to eat then go pig out, which is a bad idea. During the down time you're starving yourself you're just making it that much harder to digest all that good food.

Next time you go out to eat at a buffet, try loading up your plate with steamed vegetables along with your main entree, then go back for seconds and repeat.

Try eating fresh fruit for dessert and pass on the pie and don't drink the soda, try fresh sweetened ice tea or flavored water. These changes may take time and having that apple pie isn't as bad as it seems in moderation. Having any of the foods you love aren't bad, but having them too often and too much is. So don't overdo it and bring on the doggy bag.

ALTERNATIVES TO FRYING FOODS:

BAKING:
Is one of the simplest forms of cooking, baking your food in the oven is as easy as setting the timer and waiting for your meal. Most of the foods we love to eat fried can come as crispy and healthier in the oven. Vegetables also taste good baked and still hold some of their nutritional value as well including fries. Try baking some of your favorites in the oven like fish, chicken, or steaks.

STEWING:
Involves putting your food in flavored seasoned water and letting it cook slowly, in as little as 20 mins. Stewing your vegetables makes them soft to and meats such as ox tails become tenderer.

STIR FYING:
Is like frying your food, but with a much less volume of oil and at a faster rate of speed. Constant turning or stirring of the food is essential to prevent burning. Rice and vegetables

are usually a main ingredient in stir fried dishes with not so much meat or poultry as in normal entrees

GRILLING:

Your food is fun and it comes out tasting more favorable than fried foods. Grilling vegetables are also a more healthful treat, such as shieskabobs, with grilled pineapples, apples, etc. Seasoning or marinating your meats beforehand is recommended. Barbeques also serves as social events that the entire family and friends can enjoy. Make sure your grill heats up properly first before cooking to get the best flavor from your meats.

ALTERNATIVES TO RED MEAT

Research has shown that heavy red meat consumption increased the risk of terminal disease. The reason for this is that meat usually takes 2-3 days to digest, so when you eat it on a daily basis you're not allowing your body time to process and digest it. Lowering your intake to give your body the time to digest will improve overall health, but removing it all together from your diet would be your ultimate choice. Good luck.

Studies have also discovered that eating meat hardens blood vessels, arteries and contain meat additive that contain additional fats. Eating processed meat (Spam, hot dogs) can also in time lead, to developing Obesity and type 2 diabetes. Cutting back on how much meat you consume and eating healthier protein sources such as fish, poultry, nuts, and beans can also be good options.

FISH: is a healthy and tasty alternative to eating red meat. The health benefits of eating fish have been proven putting it high on the category of healthy foods to eat. Fish comes loaded with nutrients, protein, vitamin D, and Omega- 3 fatty acids (which helps in body and brain development, and aid in disease prevention.)

Eating fish can also lower your risk for heart disease, help prevention of Alzheimer's disease, diabetes, and even vision problems due to aging. The vitamin D you get from eating fish can bring up your levels of deficiency. Easy to prepare by baking, grilling, (remember you want to limit your intakes of fried foods to be successful) some of the best fish to eat are salmon, trout, tuna, and catfish.

CHICKEN: Chicken is so much better and healthier than red meat with less fat, less calories chicken is certainly a great, lean protein source. Just remember to remove the skin and minimize or cut out frying it. There are also health benefits from eating poultry as well. There's a reason we eat chicken soup to feel better it has been said to enhance your mood and also help in heart health.

PIZZA: When you're ordering that large pizza with the works you're sneaking on the pounds. Not only is the amount of cheese we eat fattening but also high in sodium. I recommend asking for low fat cheese and packing on the veggies. Making your own pizza in the oven is even better, that way you can control what ingredients you add and even a few healthy alternatives not normally available at your local pizzeria.

BEANS: There are many types of beans good for your daily source of protein pinto, kidney, soybeans, and navy to name a few. They don't contain any cholesterol unless they're refried beans. The healthy nutrients inside them include potassium, folate, magnesium, calcium, and vitamin B6.

REDESIGNING THE FOOD PYRAMID

Many Americans eat by this chart, some on a daily basis, which has been presumed to be a cause of obesity. We all grew up on the familiar version **breads on the bottom, fruits and veggies next, then dairies and meats, and finally fats, oils & sweets at the top.**

That well-known common version has received multiple changes. The most noticeable being the change from a pyramid to a plate (my plate) with sections for fruits, grains, vegetables and protein. The dairy is a represented in a small circle in a cup on the side.

Whole grains which are a large part of the pyramid has in fact been considered not as important to overall health as once believed. After being processed those natural benefits are eliminated. What we're left with is a minimal amount of fiber and nutritious value. Reducing your consumption should be considered. Most of the cereal we love have added sugars and food coloring and preservatives, even those one boasting of whole grain.
The fruits and veggies we eat should be fresh

and not canned or dried to reap their nutritional rewards. If you can get your fruits organic which is a little more expensive but contains less of the pesticides used in non-organic and also has a higher build of antioxidants.

One ingredient missing from the pyramid so many have lived by since its conception is water. Drinking water is essential to remain healthy. Milk is not as essential as first believed in fact the calcium we need comes in the form of vegetables like kale. Fresh fruit can provide this in the form of juicing, but drinking sweetened fruit drinks we find in the store filled with High Fructose Corn Syrup are more hurtful than helpful.

Dairy is considered an intricate part of healthy bones, and the truth is calcium comes from other sources such as broccoli, collard greens, okra, cooked spinach and turnip greens. Low fat milk is advisable, but after the pasteurization process those benefits are minimized. Drinking almond or Soy milk in my opinion make for better choices. If you eat cheese on a regular basis choose low fat cheeses.

Meat

Many Americans get their protein from red meat. While consumed lightly it can offer additional nutrients like iron, zinc, niacin, and riboflavin, Seafood, and poultry fall in this category and can be better choices, Also protein can also be found in seeds, beans, nuts, fish and poultry.

Remember if you choose meat cut back on eating processed meats like bacon, which can be high in fat and salt. Choose lean meat trimmed of excess fat and be sure to remove the skin from your chicken. Minimize your portions and allow the food to digest properly (somewhere between **24-72 hours**) before stuffing yourself some more. Make sure to add lots of whole grains and lots of vegetables to your plate.

Here's a few healthy dinner recipes you can try to add some variety to the dinner table.

Grilled Lemon Pepper Chicken
4-6 large chicken breasts (skinless)
1 sliced lemon
1 tablespoon of virgin olive oil
Seasoning salt to taste
1 sliced green or red pepper

¼ teaspoon of black pepper
1 teaspoon oregano

Directions
1. Pre heat grill until nice and hot spray on some Pam or nonstick spray or use aluminum foil to prevent burning.

2 Place chicken and pepper on grill.

3. Let cook, occasionally flipping until well-cooked squeeze some lemon juice on top, remove and serve,

Salmon Salad
1 Salmon Fillet
1 Bell Pepper
½ cup water
1 tomato
¼ fresh parsley
3 tablespoon reduced fat mayonnaise
1 cup chopped celery
1/8 teaspoon ground black pepper
8 leaves lettuce
1 (16 ounce) package elbow macaroni
2 ripe tomatoes, diced
4 green onions, chopped

2 dill pickles, diced
½ cup mayonnaise
salt and pepper to taste

Directions
1. Pre heat oven to 400 degrees place salmon on nonstick pan, let bake for 15 minutes until done Cut the salmon into small sections place in bowl, removing the skin or bones.
2. In a small bowl combine the mayonnaise, onions, pickles, tomatoes, celery, and pepper. Mix well and then toss in the salmon.
Bring a large pot of water to a boil. Add pasta and cook for 8 to 10 minutes or until ready and soft; drain water. Let cool.

3. Mix pasta in small bowl and mix well. Serve over fresh lettuce.

Clam Chowder
2 cups of peeled cube potatoes
3 (6 ounce can of canned chopped clams
1 cup minced onion
1 cup diced celery
1 garlic
1 cup diced carrots
1 cup of water

2   bottles of clam juice
1/3 cup of all-purpose flour
3/4 cup butter
½ tablespoon of salt
3 (6.5 ounce) cans minced clams
 1 quart half-and-half cream
 ground black pepper to seasoning

Directions

1. Drain juice from clams into a large skillet over the onions, celery, potatoes and carrots. Add water to cover, and cook over medium heat until tender.

2. Meanwhile, in a large, heavy saucepan, melt the butter over medium heat. Whisk in flour until smooth. Whisk in cream and stir constantly until thick and smooth. Stir in vegetables and clam juice. Heat through, but do not boil.

3. Stir in clams just before serving. If they cook too much they will get tough. When clams are heated through, stir and season with salt and pepper.

Garlic Lemon Lamb Chops

4 loin lamb chops freshly cut
2 garlic cloves
3 tablespoons water
¼ cup of fresh parsley
pinch of dried thyme
3 tablespoons extra-virgin olive oil
2 tablespoons fresh lemon juice
½ teaspoon of fine ground red pepper
½ teaspoon salt
¼ teaspoon fresh-ground black pepper

Directions

1. Season the lamb with salt and pepper and light thyme.
2. Heat the olive oil in a large skillet.
3. Add lamb chops and garlic and cook slowly over high heat until the chops are brown well on one bottom side, about 3 ½ minutes.
4. Flip lamb chops and cook until the chops are brown,
5. Set lamb chops to plates, leaving the garlic in the skillet.
6. Add the water, lemon juice, parsley and ground red pepper to the pan and simmer until hot, about 1 ½ minute. Baste the garlic sauce over the lamb chops and serve.

Pineapple Chicken

Ingredients
½ cup barbecue sauce
½ cup orange juice
¼ cup packed brown sugar
2 tablespoons canola oil
2 tablespoons all-purpose flour
¼ teaspoon salt, optional
4 boneless skinless chicken breast halves (1 pound)
1 can (8 ounces) pineapple rings in natural juice, drained
1 ½ teaspoons ground ginger
¼ up honey
¼ cup Dijon mustard
1/8 teaspoon pepper
2 garlic cloves, minced

Directions
1. Sprinkle chicken with salt and pepper.
2. In a skillet, brown chicken in oil. Meanwhile, drain pineapple,
3. Cut pineapple rings in half and set aside reserving the juice.
4. In a large saucepan, combine barbecue sauce, orange juice, brown sugar, canola oil, flour until creamy. Bring to a boil; reduce heat and simmer

for 2 ½/ minutes, occasionally stirring.
5. Combine mustard, honey, garlic and remaining pineapple juice; mix well.
Remove chicken and keep warm.
Serve over hot cooked rice.
Top with pineapple and sauce to taste.

Vegetable Lasagna

1 (16 ounce) package lasagna noodles
1 pound fresh mushrooms, sliced
3/4 cup chopped onion
3 cloves garlic, minced
2 (26 ounce) jars pasta sauce
1 (15 ounce) container part-skim ricotta cheese
4 cups shredded mozzarella cheese
2 Eggs Large
½ cup grated Parmesan cheese
12 lasagna noodles
2 tablespoons virgin olive oil
3 heads chopped fresh broccoli,
2 carrots, thinly sliced
1 large onion, chopped
2 green bell peppers, chopped
2 small zucchini, sliced
½ cup all-purpose flour
3 cups milk
½ teaspoon salt

½ teaspoon pepper

1 (10 ounce) package frozen chopped spinach, thawed

1 cup tomato sauce

Directions

1. Preheat oven to 375 degrees F. spray a 9x12-inch baking dish with nonstick spray.

2. Bring a large pot of water to a boil. Add lasagna noodles and cook for 8 to 10 minutes or until ready, drain in strainer.

3. Heat oil in a large skillet over medium heat. When oil is hot add carrots, broccoli, bell peppers, onions, zucchini and garlic. Simmer for 8 minutes; put aside.

4. Place flour in a medium saucepan and gradually mix in milk until well blended. Bring to a boil over medium heat. Cook 5 minutes, until thick, stirring often. Stir in ½ cup Parmesan cheese, salt and pepper; cook for 1 minute, stirring. Remove from heat; add spinach. Take ½ cup spinach mix. In a small bowl, combine cottage and ricotta cheeses; stir well.

5. Spread about ½ cup of spinach mixture in the bottom of the prepared pan. Layer lasagna noodles, ricotta mixture, vegetables, spinach

mixture, tomato sauce and 2 cups mozzarella cheese, ending with lasagna noodles. Top with spinach mixture you put to the side, ½ cup mozzarella cheese and ¼ cup Parmesan cheese.

6. Bake in preheated oven for 35- 40 minutes, or until lightly browned on top. Cool for approximately 10 minutes before serving.

Step 6

THE PLAN

TIPS
Eating Salad can be a good way to slim down, but pouring on the ranch only boosts your calorie intake up, so switching to vinaigrette is recommended. Chicken is essentially a good choice, but removing the skin or ordering it grilled is your best bet. Cutting back on the cheese, which can be an addictive food will lower the calories on all your meals, try to do without it if you can and see the dramatic changes you can make simply by doing so.

Reducing the amount of sauce you dress your meals up with, whether it be a burger or a salad will also cut back on the calories and fat in a major way. Also loading your sandwich with fresh healthy veggies like lettuce, tomato, spinach, or even nuts will give you the roughage you need to stay full and less hungry. And remember cutting out the High Fructose Corn Syrup sodas is a big step on the road to the new you.

HOW TO ORDER HEALTHY
Eating healthy doesn't have to mean eating lettuce and carrots for lunch, when we look at the menu to order we automatically have a set of programmed choices that we usually go for subconsciously and stick by it. Some restaurants now offer the calorie count on their menus making the choice a little easier.

The main foods you want to cut back or out altogether are the ones deep fried and smothered in cheese, which is mostly fat. For instance eating a pizza with the works, when you add all the pepperoni, ham, ground beef and Italian sausage etc. on top of the cheese it's a belly-buster. Ordering your Pizza vegetarian style is a better choice with no extra cheese or butter.

Okay time to go to work, I suggest easing into plan probably by picking your favorite item of any one week and trying that first just to throw off any craving you may feel, after that I would suggest going by the plan. I suggest you try a smoothie or freshly squeezed juice from my recipes to start off your day. Any breakfast you eat should be light, added to the juice.

So are you ready to get healthier and still eat what you love? Now remember this is a plan, adding to it on the heavy side could set you back so keep within the limits and allow your body time to adjust to the changes in your diet.

Around 500 calories or less a day for lunch is the goal.

LUNCH MENU

Week 1:

McDonald's: Monday	Fruit n Yogurt Parfait	Artisan Grilled Chicken
Calories	380	380
Total Fat	2g	6g
Saturated Fat	1g	1.5g
Cholesterol	5mg	80mg
Sodium	80mg	930mg
Carbs	30g	43g
Fiber	1g	3g
Sugars	23g	11g
Protein	4g	32g

Wendy's: Tuesday Small Chili			
Calories	180	Carbs	20g
Total Fat	5g	Fibers	4g
Saturated Fat	2g	Sugars	5g
Cholesterol	30mg	Protein	13g
Sodium	790mg	N/A	N/A

Burger King: Wed	Whopper Jr.
Calories	310
Total Fat	16
Saturated Fat	4.5g
Cholesterol	25mg
Sodium	460mg
Carbs	27g

Fiber	1g
Sugars	7g
Protein	9g
Subway: Thursday	**Turkey Breast Sub**
Calories	330
Total Fat	9g
Saturated Fat	2g
Cholesterol	5mg
Sodium	20mg
Carbs	46g
Fiber	5g
Sugars	7g
Protein	18g
McDonald's: Friday	**Sante Fe Veggie Wrap**
Calories	216
Total Fat	24g
Saturated Fat	6g
Cholesterol	20mg
Sodium	980mg
Carbs	56g
Fiber	10g
Sugars	7g
Protein	15g

Week 2:

Burger King: Mon	**Angus Steak Burger**
Calories	280
Total Fat	22g
Saturated Fat	8g

Cholesterol	180mg
Sodium	1190mg
Carbs	59g
Fiber	3g
Sugars	13g
Protein	33g
Burger King: Tues	**Veggie Burger**
Calories	390
Total Fat	1g
Saturated Fat	8g
Cholesterol	0mg
Sodium	840mg
Carbs	43g
Fiber	5g
Sugars	19g
Protein	21g
Burger King: Wed	**BK Fish Fillet Sandwich**
Calories	520
Total Fat	30g
Saturated Fat	8g
Cholesterol	55mg
Sodium	840mg
Carbs	44g
Fiber	2g
Sugars	4g
Protein	18g

Wendy's: Thursday	Grilled Chicken Classic
Calories	360
Total Fat	9g
Saturated Fat	2g
Cholesterol	65mg
Sodium	820mg
Carbs	42g
Fiber	3g
Sugars	8g
Protein	28g
Arby's: Friday	Roast Beef Deli
Calories	320
Total Fat	13g
Saturated Fat	3g
Cholesterol	45mg
Sodium	950mg
Carbs	34g
Fiber	2g
Sugars	5g
Protein	21g

Week 3:

McDonald's: Monday	Mc Artesian
Calories	380
Total Fat	22g
Saturated Fat	8g
Cholesterol	180mg
Sodium	1190mg
Carbs	59g

Fiber	3g
Sugars	13g
Protein	33g

Wendy's: Tuesday	Small Chili	Baked Potato (light sour cream)
Calories	170	310
Total Fat	5g	2.5g
Saturated Fat	2g	1.5g
Cholesterol	35mg	10mg
Sodium	780mg	35mg
Carbs	16g	63g
Fiber	4g	3g
Sugars	6g	4g
Protein	33g	8g

Taco Bell: Wednesday	Burrito Supreme Steak
Calories	390
Total Fat	16g
Saturated Fat	7g
Cholesterol	35mg
Sodium	1260mg
Carbs	50g
Fiber	6g
Sugars	5g
Protein	19g

Wendy's: Thursday	Asian Cashew Chicken
Calories	380
Total Fat	10g
Saturated Fat	1.5g

Cholesterol	45mg
Sodium	520mg
Carbs	20g
Fiber	4g
Sugars	0g
Protein	20g
Arby's: Friday	**Grand Turkey Club**
Calories	380
Total Fat	24g
Saturated Fat	7g
Cholesterol	0mg
Sodium	1610mg
Carbs	37g
Fiber	2g
Sugars	9g
Protein	30g

Week 4:

Subway: Monday	**6" Veggie Delite**
Calories	230
Total Fat	19g
Saturated Fat	3.5g
Cholesterol	40mg
Sodium	650mg
Carbs	15g
Fiber	1g
Sugars	1g
Protein	11g

McDonald's: Tuesday	Premium Southwest Salad with Grilled Chicken
Calories	350
Total Fat	12g
Saturated Fat	4.5g
Cholesterol	100mg
Sodium	1027mg
Carbs	29g
Fiber	6.7g
Sugars	10g
Protein	36g
Wendy's: Wednesday	Premium Cod Filet
Calories	510
Total Fat	19g
Saturated Fat	3.5g
Cholesterol	40mg
Sodium	650mg
Carbs	15g
Fiber	1g
Sugars	1g
Protein	11g
Taco Bell: Thursday	Chicken Rancho Taco (Fresco)
Calories	240
Total Fat	4g
Saturated Fat	1g
Cholesterol	25mg
Sodium	710mg

Carbs	22g
Fiber	3g
Sugars	12g
Protein	
Arby's: Friday	**Southwest Grilled Chicken Wrap (light sauce)**
Calories	564
Total Fat	34g
Saturated Fat	10g
Cholesterol	77mg
Sodium	1606mg
Carbs	41g
Fiber	3g
Sugars	3g
Protein	31g

This Plan is designed to get you in the habit of ordering healthy when you eat on the go. These weekly plans are something you can mix and match as time goes on to your taste. But Remember the math still stands and so does the food for fuel rule. If you add to the menu on the heavy side including packing on the special sauces then you can expect to slowly add on the pounds.

No one knows your body like you, so as you adjust to your new diet you'll be able to change it up a little through the weeks. As time goes on hopefully you'll be able to pick and choose healthy items of your choice while still eating your favorites just not as much. This plan will give you results if you follow the tips and changes outlined in this book. I won't make any promises because it all comes down to commitment and determination. The trick is learning to love to eat healthier foods that still have a familiar taste that we crave without the unhealthy health risk. The real key is utilizing you snacking and keeping your cravings to a minimal. When you get hungry don't hold off and try to make it to lunch because you'll go pass you daily limits and overeat. Having a light healthy snack will cure those hunger pangs and keep you on the right track.

Don't forget that hunger can be mistaken with thirst, drinking water can fill those gaps throughout the day. When you start to see results such as feeling more energetic and less sluggish, less hungry throughout the day and the pounds start rolling away, then you'll know that you're making a smooth adjustment.

HITTING THE GYM

Working out doesn't always have to mean going out to the gym. With the countless number of home gyms available out there, you can bring the gym home to you. Exercise equipment like Treadmills, Stair Steppers and Stationary Bikes can fit easily inside your home making them very convenient. With prices ranging upwards to as much as $3000, make sure to shop around first before settling in on a particular machine to purchase. Workout videos and music can help incorporate dance moves into your exercise routines to add some variety to your workout. Exercise should be fun. Use headphones and create yourself a personal workout playlist of adrenaline pumping tunes.

Having a daily workout routine has major health advantages. It can also help in relieving stress, anxiety and even depression. Studies have proven that being physically inactive is the major cause of weight gain. So of naturally exercise is the complete polar opposite. Cutting back on your calorie intake is a big key, but those calories will be cut a lot faster with a steady exercise routine. Building muscle mass can help maximize in fat burning by keeping your metabolism revved up. As we increase in age we naturally lose some of our strength and muscle mass decreases. In time you'll find your energy levels increasing and that sluggish feeling you get from CF (chronic fatigue syndrome) start to evaporate. Swimming, dancing, running and even walking are all great exercises to aid in fat burning.

WEIGHT LOSS PROGRAMS

Diets designed by experts and hundreds of tasty nutritious entrees on their menus, weight loss programs seem like a sure thing when it comes to losing weight. Some weight loss programs offer food delivery, healthy items like protein bars, shakes, and snacks with charts and personal advisers available. However, these plans aren't designed for everyone including pregnant women, people with allergies to certain foods or children. By eating every 2-3 hours, snacking and eating smaller more well balanced portions, this helps promote weight loss and keeps your metabolism going, which is key to giving a boost to weight loss. Remember to check with your doctor or physicians first before starting any weight loss programs, if you have any prior health conditions or concerns.

Here are some of the best programs to choose from to help you with losing weight

Nutrisystem
One of the most popular around it offers meals low in unhealthy fats and high in fiber and lean protein for breakfast, lunch, and dinner with healthy snacks available to order. Vegetarian options are available on the 160+ items offered on their menu, with special programs for people with diabetes. The prices can range from $9 to $11 per meal and between $235 to $275 a month or more.

Jenny Craig
Operating since 1991 this program offers 100+ low calorie prepackaged foods, weight loss support in the form of a one on one consultant to help you lose weight and an exercise plan to keep in shape. Prices range between $140 to $156 a week for food.

South Beach Diet
This program offers foods low in carbs, high in protein and healthy fat. Their items can help

change your eating habits by restricting bad carbs (bread, rice, pastas, alcohol, certain fruits and fruit juices) and promoting exercise. As you gradually lose weight you can incorporate some of those forbidden foods back into your diet. It even offers an app you can download to your phone to keep track with meals, and weight loss. Also they can assign you a health counselor who you can contact through phone, email or online. Prices range between $230.00 $340.00 a month.

Bistro MD

Created by doctors and registered dieticians with food prepared by professional chefs, they offer tasty nutritious meals in their diet program with a wide variety of up to 150 meals that are not processed. Their dishes are full of protein with a nice size serving of vegetables along with snacks to leave you satisfied and full. With a diet program created by doctors this makes the selections you choose from easier to coincide with your specific needs. Prices can range from $145 to $ 180 per week, not including delivery fees.

PREGNANCY

Gaining a little weight during and after pregnancy is normal for women. Breastfeeding, exercise and eating healthy meals can help with shedding those extra pounds. Changing your diet during your pregnancy to healthier selections is very beneficial to you and your growing baby. Try cutting back on the fried foods, the junk food, and eating more fruits and vegetables. Switching flavored water for carbonated soft drinks (soda pop) is another good option.

Simple task such as walking, jogging or even tending to your garden can be effective with helping with weight loss. Swimming, yoga and riding a stationary exercise bike are also good. Some exercises like sit- ups could possibly be harmful to your baby, so remember to always talk with your doctor before beginning on which exercises to do during your pregnancy.

WEIGHT LOSS PILL

Although a lot of them have been proven to not live up to their promises, some natural dietary supplements can boost your metabolism helping to reduce cravings while aiding in fat loss and increasing muscle mass. Remember there is no supernatural way of losing weight, changing to a more balanced diet and making lifestyle changes are the main ingredients to this process. With some weight loss pills containing ingredients that are banned by the FDA, always make sure you check with your doctor or physician beforehand before using any dietary supplements.

WEIGHT LOSS SURGERY
Bariatric surgery has been considered a final alternative to exercise and dietary changes. The prices can range from $14,000 upwards to $20,000 or more. Gastric bypass surgery is the most common practice in which the digestive system is limited to how much you can eat. Due to some serious overweight health conditions, certain qualifications must be met beforehand. After the surgery lifestyle changes must be applied to your diet. As with any other serious surgical procedure there's the risk of complications and side effects. **DINING AT HOME**

Preparing your own food at home is a good way to save money, but eating healthy on a budget can prove to be a challenge. There's no denying that saving money can dictate what does and doesn't go into the refrigerator. The truth is you can still eat healthy and also stay within your grocery budget. Planning ahead for the upcoming week can be a good way to shorten your grocery list. Instead of loading up for the entire month, try shopping weekly or bi-weekly. Try resisting the temptation to pick up items that are not on your grocery list. These impulsive selections can quickly send you over your budget. Look to purchase whole foods such as produce (from a fruit market if one is available in your area), unsalted nuts, seeds, beans, whole grain rice and oats. Avoid over processed foods typically found in the inner aisles of the store. Doing so will help in saving you tons of money. Remember to pick up a few healthy snacks for work to reduce those trips to the vending machines at work. (pretzels, unsalted almonds, sun flower kernels, granola bars etc.) Cutting back on and purchasing less meat will help both with weight loss and also your budget.

Here are a few more easy entrees and some healthy desserts for you to try out

Barbecue Vegan Pizza

Trader Joe's Cauliflower Pizza Crust
3/4 cup BBQ sauce
1 sliced red or yellow bell pepper (seeds and stem removed)
1 ½ cup of fresh mushrooms
1 cup sliced zucchini
1 onion peeled and sliced
1 cup diced tomatoes
1 cup shredded mozzarella
10 oz sliced baked or grilled vegan chicken strips
2 tbls of olive oil
*add or replace with vegetables of your choice.

Directions

1. Preheat oven to 375 degrees F (190 degrees C).
2. Add one tablespoon of oil to baking sheet.
3. Spread around the place where the pizza dough will go.
4. Place pizza unfrozen dough on the baking sheet then spread equal amounts of BBQ sauce over the dough.
5. Sprinkle with half of the mozzarella cheese. Top with bell pepper, zucchini, onions, mushroom and fresh tomatoes (or replace with

any other veggies of your choice) Sprinkle the remaining cheese over top.
6. Place the prepped pizza in the oven
7. Bake for 25- 30 minutes or until crust is golden brown and dough is cooked through.
8. After remove the pizza from the oven. Let cool then slice and eat.

Turkey Tacos

1 teaspoon olive oil
2 tablespoons premium Taco Seasoning
3 cloves garlic minced
1 pound ground turkey
1 (8 ounce) can tomato sauce
1 teaspoon brown sugar
Salt and black pepper (seasoned to taste)
Corn tortillas
Directions

1. Heat oil in a large skillet over medium-high heat. Add onion and cook until softened, (5 minutes or so)
2. Add taco seasoning, garlic, stir for about 30 seconds.
3. Add ground turkey and cook, stir occasionally, until cooked. Stir in tomato sauce and brown sugar. Cook until thickened, about 5

minutes. Season to taste with salt and pepper.

Divide filling evenly among tortillas and serve with healthy garnishes such as shredded lettuce, tomato, onions, salsa or guacamole. Serve and enjoy.

Turkey Chili
2 teaspoons olive oil
1 onion, chopped
3 garlic cloves, minced
1 medium red bell pepper, chopped
1 jalapeno pepper, cored, deveined and finely chopped
1 pound extra lean ground turkey or chicken
4 tablespoons of chili powder
2 teaspoons ground cumin
1 teaspoon dried oregano
1/4 teaspoon cayenne pepper
½ teaspoon salt, plus more to taste
1 (28-ounce) can diced tomatoes or crushed tomatoes
1 1/4 cups fresh or canned chicken broth
2 (15 oz) cans dark red kidney beans, rinsed and drained
1 (15 oz) can sweet corn, rinsed and drained
add salt and ground black pepper (seasoned to taste)

Directions

1. Place oil in a large pot and place over medium high heat.
2. Add in onion, garlic and red pepper and sauté for 5-7 minutes, stirring frequently.
3. Next add in ground turkey and break up the meat; cooking until no longer pink.
4. Next add in chili powder, cumin, oregano, cayenne pepper and salt; stir for about 20 seconds.
5. Next add in tomatoes, chicken broth, kidney beans and corn.
6. Bring to a boil, then reduce heat and simmer for 30-45 minutes or until chili thickens and flavors come together.

(optional)
top with fat free shredded cheddar cheese
sour cream

Stuffed Pepper

2 yellow bell peppers
1 (8 ounce) can natural tomato sauce
1 tablespoon Worcestershire sauce
salt and ground black pepper to taste
1 (8 ounce) can natural tomato sauce

1 teaspoon Italian seasoning
1/4 cup grated Parmesan cheese, optional

Directions

1. Preheat oven to 350 degrees F (175 degrees C).
2. Bring brown rice and water to a boil in a saucepan. Reduce heat to medium-low, cover, and simmer until rice is tender and liquid has been absorbed, 45 to 50 minutes.
3. Cook and stir beef, garlic, and onion in a skillet over medium heat until meat is evenly browned and onion is softened, about 5 minutes.
4. Remove and discard the tops, seeds, and membranes of the green, red, and yellow bell peppers. Arrange peppers in a baking dish with the hollowed sides facing upward. Slice the bottoms off the peppers if necessary so that they stand upright.
5. Mix the browned beef, cooked rice, 1 can tomato sauce, Worcestershire sauce, salt, and pepper in a bowl. Spoon an equal amount of the mixture into each hollowed pepper. Mix the remaining tomato sauce and Italian seasoning in a bowl, and pour over the stuffed peppers.
6. Bake in the preheated oven, basting with sauce every 15 minutes, until the peppers are

tender, about 1 hour. Sprinkle the peppers with grated Parmesan cheese after baking.

Honey Baked Salmon

1/4 cup honey
3 cloves garlic, minced
1 tablespoon extra-virgin olive oil
1 tsp red pepper flakes
1 tablespoon fresh thyme leaves
Kosher salt and freshly ground pepper seasoned to taste
2 pounds of salmon fillets
1 tbsp lemon juice

Directions

1. Preheat oven to 375 degrees F. Line a baking sheet with foil.
2. In a small bowl, mix together the honey, lemon juice, thyme, olive oil and red pepper flakes.
3. Place salmon onto prepared baking sheet with the skin facing up and fold up all the sides of the foil.
4. Spoon the honey mixture on top of the salmon. Fold the sides of the foil over the top of the salmon, covering it closed.

5. Season with salt and pepper to taste

6. Bake for about 20 minutes or until fully cooked through.

7. Add the honey sauce over the top of the salmon.

8. Serve and enjoy.

Peanut Butter Rice Crispy Treats

3 tbsp butter
½ cup honey
½ cup creamy peanut butter
4 ¾ cups Rice Krispies cereal

Directions

1. Coat a 13 x 9 pan dish with nonstick cooking spray.
2. In a sauce pan, melt the butter with the heat on low. Be careful, not to burn the butter.
3. With the heat still on low add in the honey and the peanut butter.
4. Keep stirring make sure the peanut butter doesn't burn, stir the mixture for 5 minutes.
5. Add in the cereal, making sure to cover the cereal up good
6. Pour mixture into prepared pan and even out with a spatula.

7. Let cool or put in the refrigerator.
8. Slice and serve.

Zucchini Brownies

2 cups shredded zucchini
1 ½ tsp baking soda
1 tsp salt
½ cup of coconut oil
1 tsp pure vanilla extract
1 large egg
1/4 cup cocoa powder
1 cup dark chocolate chips
1 ½ cups whole wheat flour

Directions

1. Preheat the oven to 350. Line a 9×9 inch baking dish with parchment paper. Shred the zucchini, (use a grater if you have one) do not peel it.
2. Place the coconut oil and ½ cup of the dark chocolate chips in a small nonstick frying pan over a medium heat and let melt. Once they have melted remove the pan from heat.
3. Add the whole wheat flour, cocoa powder, baking soda, and salt to a large bowl then mix together.

4. In a medium bowl mix together the eggs, grated zucchini, coconut oil and vanilla.
5. Once the chocolate has cooled slightly, add it to the bowl with the eggs and mix together. Pour this into the bowl with the whole wheat flour and mix together. Stir in the remaining ½ cup of dark chocolate chips.
6. Pour the brownie batter into the prepared baking dish and spread it around the pan with a spatula.
7. Bake in the oven for 20 to 30 minutes (stick a fork in it to make sure it's done) then remove the pan from the oven and let it sit for 5-10 minutes or until cool. Lift the brownies out of the pan using the parchment paper to make sure that they've cool off.
8. Cut them into a 12 -16 pieces. Serve.

FROZEN DINNERS

TV dinners or frozen dinners have been a popular alternative to cooking at home since 1953. A large variety of choices can now be found in the frozen food aisle of your local grocery store. With a wide range of meals from traditional dinners like Baked Chicken, Turkey dinners, Asian cuisines, Vegetarian, non GMO meals and new selections being offered routinely there's unquestionably something there for everyone.

Keep aware of the nutritional value by checking out the charts and ingredients on the side panel. Light frozen dinners can contain under 300 calories and usually no more than 8 grams of fat. Keep that in mind when you're making your selections. Eating frozen meals with a low calorie count can help with weight loss, but some people may not feel full from them and find themselves snacking in between meals even more. Be mindful of this when adjusting to your new lifestyle changes.

Some healthy selections

Lean Cuisine Butternut Squash Ravioli
(260 calories, 7 grams of fat)

Smart Ones Lemon Herb Chicken Picatta
(210 Calories, 3 grams of fat)

Lean Cuisine Meatloaf and Mashed Potatoes
(230 calories, 6 grams of fat)

Lean Cuisine Herb Roasted Chicken
(170 calories, 4 grams of fat)

Michelina's Lean Gourmet Chicken Alfredo Florentine
(270 calories, 3 grams of fat)

Healthy Choice Mushroom Roasted Beef
(280 calories, 3 grams of fat)

Seeds of Change Chicken Teriyaki
(300 calories, 3 ½ grams of fat)

Smart Ones: Tuna Noodle Casserole
(250 calories, 3 grams of fat)

Saffron Road: Chickem Tiki Massala
(280 calories, 3 grams of fat)

DINING OUT

Going out to eat is both a treat for the entire family. Having other people prepare your meals is convenient and saves you lots of time. With the wide variety of restaurants available out there offering various different types of delicious food to choose from, the selections are sure to keep you interested. Healthy choices are available so check out some of the online menus of your favorites to make sure they offer healthy items to your liking. Remember to order your food grilled, roasted, or broiled. If a salad bar is available try making your own salad, if one is not make sure to order it with light dressing and light cheese.

FAMILY BUFFET

You might say to yourself that All-You-Can Eat and losing weight just don't go together. With endless entrees available the urge to go back for seconds, thirds and so on. The key to it is not overdoing it you can have a little of your favorites, but not a lot. Before you start piling up your plate with some of your favorites check out your options.

Start your meal with a small salad light on the dressing or a cup of warm soup to curb your appetite. Switching the sweets for fresh fruit is a good alternative for dessert. Drinking a lot of water will be much better than hitting the soda fountain. If you can sweeting it up with splashes of fresh fruit for some flavor.

Try passing on the fried foods including the French Fries. Avoid the gravy and thick sauces. Go easy on the meat selections and go for the grilled or baked choices. Don't stuff your face enjoy your food! Take time to let your food digest properly before rushing off for seconds.

With more than one million restaurants in the United States to choose from, there's an endless selection of healthy cuisines out there to try. And now most even offer online ordering which gives you the luxury of having your food prepared before you even get there

Here's a healthy selections of ethnic cuisines to try

Chinese

Chinese food is a healthy choice when you load up on the vegetables which will give you plenty of fiber. Take heed to limiting your intake of white rice and noodles. Order your selections with lean meat, skinless chicken, fish or tofu. Pass on the fatty cuts of beef and pork and deep fried chicken, eggrolls and fried wontons. Try ordering your meal steamed, stir fried in light oil, boiled, or broiled.

A few healthy selections:

Moo Goo Gai Pan (chicken & vegetables)
168 calories 6 grams of fat
Beef and Broccoli
150 calories 7 grams of fat
Chop Suey (with your choice of meat or poultry)
336 calories 17 grams of fat
Moo Shu Chicken (with light sauce)
273 calories 18 grams of fat
Wonton Soup
71 calories .06 grams of fat

Greek

Greek food offers foods lean on meat. Prepared with healthy ingredients like olive oil, fresh fruits, vegetables such as garlic, tomatoes, spinach and also nuts. With foods rich in antioxidants the Mediterranean diet can help in lowering the risk of heart disease, type 2 diabetes, obesity, and cancer. Try some of their Greek Yogurt, it's packed with protein, potassium, calcium and probiotics which can help your immune system. Natural energy providing Vitamin B12, which helps with forming red blood cells, and brain activity. Some of the healthier dishes include:

Hummus
  25 calories 1.5 grams of fat
Melitzanosalata (Eggplant salad)
  130 calories 4 grams of fat
Avgloemono (chicken and pasta soup)
  341 calories 9 grams of fat
Gigante Plaki (white beans in tomato soup)
  320 calories 16 grams of fat
Chicken Souvlaki (chicken grilled on a skewer)
260 calories   8 grams of fat

Indian

Indian food offers meals low in fat that include a variety of spices, fruits, vegetables, rice, and lean meats. Choose vegetable based sauces over the creamy blends, chicken and seafood over beef or lamb and pass on the fried foods like samosas and the fry breads also. Order you meats Tandoori (oven grilled) or steamed. Avoid eating rice and if you do eat smaller helpings.

A few healthy selections:

Roti Bread (whole wheat)
122 calories 19 grams of fat
Tandoori Chicken or Fish
263 calories 12 grams of fat
Chana Masala (chickpea curry)
281 calories 16 grams from fat
Dal (stew)
74 calories 1.8 grams of fat
Kokum Kadhi
125 calories 12 grams of fat

Italian

Italian cuisine is considered to be a part of the Mediterranean diet, with ingredients that include fresh vegetables like tomatoes, garlic, olive oil, beans, and leafy greens such as spinach. Italian restaurants offer dishes low in calories and filled with nutritional benefits. This also includes foods rich in fiber like whole grain breads and pastas that can help in maintaining or reducing weight. If you can replace the butter on your bread with olive oil which is much healthier and be sure to limit the amount of cheese and creamy sauces added to your meal, a big step in reducing calories.

Try some of these dishes out:

Chicken Cacciatoi
233 calories 7 grams of fat
Caprese Salad (tomatoes, white mozzarella, basil
& olive oil) *220 calories 17 grams of fat*
Thin crust Veggie Pizza
173 calories 7 grams of fat (per slice)
Spaghetti Marinara
392 calories 22 grams of fat

Japanese

With a diet that includes more fish than meat Japanese cuisines are packed with a wide range of fruits and vegetables steamed or stir fried. Try passing on the Agemono, Tempura or Tankatsu, which are all deep fried in oil. Low in calories Japanese food is definitely considered to be one of the healthier choices when dining out. Of course when you're talking about Japanese dishes you can't forget the sushi (raw fish), which contain Omega-3 fatty acids that help with cardiovascular health and is also low in calories.

Recommendations:

Hot Tea
2 calories 0 grams of fat
Salmon Avocado Roll
329 calories 15 grams of fat
Udon (noodles)
208 calories 0 grams of fat
Gyoza (grilled dumpling)
240 calories 9 grams of fat
Miso Sui Soup
59 calories 3 grams of fat
Fresh Sushi or Sashimi
304 calories 8 grams of fat

Mediterranean

The Mediterranean diet is low in meat with large helpings of fruits, vegetables, fish, nuts, whole grains and olive oil. Delicious fish dishes like Salmon, Tuna, and Mackerel offer Omega-3 fatty acids that improve eye and brain function, while being beneficial to your overall heart health lowering your risk for certain diseases.

Healthy Selections:

Hummus
25 calories 1.5 grams of fat

Grilled Fish
225 calories 5 grams of fat
Greek Chicken Salad (with light dressing)
360 calories 19 grams of fat
Grilled Kabobs
276 calories 6 grams of fat
Grilled seafood with sautéed vegetables

Mexican

Mexican food at first glance doesn't exactly come across as a healthy choice. The trick is cutting back on all the cheese, choosing soft tacos over hard taco shells (which are fried in oil), and getting your meals grilled instead of fried. Replacing the sour cream with salsa is a very healthy option. Try to avoid eating the chips and salsa before your meals ready and avoid foods saturated in cheese like Chimichangas, Queso and some Burritos. Remember not to pour on the extra sauce.

Some suggested dishes to try include:
Grilled Chicken Fajitas
330 calories 16 grams of fat
Grilled Steak
293 calories 13 grams of fat
Soft Corn Tortilla Tacos (light sauce, light cheese)

260 calories 5 grams of fat
Tortilla Soup
320 calories 15 grams of fat

Thai

Thai food is very healthy, filled with intense flavors and doesn't depend so much on fats or meats. Among the spices and flavors that make Thai a stand out are turmeric, coriander, ginger, lemongrass, and chili peppers. These can offer you the health benefits of a boosted immune system. When ordering look for seafood meals and meals with lightly cooked vegetables. Pass on the fried foods like Rice or Spring Rolls, and limit eating any Coconut Milk made dishes.

Healthy Selections:

Tom Yum Goong (hot and sour soup with shrimp)
180 calories 3 grams of fat
Kaeng Liang (vegetable soup thai style)
138 calories   grams of fat
Khao Man Gai (chicken and rice)
274 calories 8 grams of fat
Som Tam (papaya salad)
124 calories 5 grams of fat

Step 7

STICKING TO THE PLAN

Okay there you have it the plan and guide to self-change. So do you believe in yourself? Are you ready to make the commitment necessary to see yourself through to the end and meet the new you? In everything we do the most important part is the follow through, that ability to take ourselves to the finish. Get things done. Whether it be swinging a golf club or completing the plan. Starting is only the beginning, but making it to the end is what counts and determines what kind of person you are, a beginner of a finisher, a winner or a quitter.

Remember this is not a magic book with secret spells, just honest information and facts to help aid you on your journey to a healthier lifestyle. Every morning when you wake up you'll ask yourself, will I give in or will I go on. I'm hoping the answer is to continue with the plan, remember only you know your body and adjusting times can take longer for some people than others. There's no time limit on weight loss, it's a journey not a destination and journeys take time to prepare for. The cravings are going to come hard and fast and constant, like a child craving attention. In other words you' 'all have to make a decision, *give in or go on*. Remember the water solution and utilizing your snacking.

I believe in all of you, otherwise I wouldn't have bothered writing this book. Remember we're a team, together we'll get through this and live fuller, healthier, well balanced lives. So let's get going down the road to success and before you know it your body will be well adjusted to your new diet, and you'll be on your way to living a healthier lifestyle.

Index

Alcohol, 44, 80;
Alternatives, 17, 25-27, 37, 39, 50-53, 82, 93, 96;
Americans, that eat fast food 1, 3, 10, 21, 22, 44, 54, 56;
Antioxidant, 19, 20, 26, 55, 98;
ARBY's, 9, 71, 73, 75;
Apples, 40-43, 46, 49, 51;
Arteries, 2, 52;
Artificial, 44, 45;
Aspartame, 45;
Attitude,
    staying positive 14;
Baked Potato, 22, 45;
    Wendy's 3, 10, 22, 72;
Baking, 45, 50, 52, 62;
Bananas, 38, 40;
Barbeque, 51, 64;
Beans, 19, 52, 53, 56, 98, 100;
    baked 11;

Beet, 43;
Beverages, 44-45;
Bike, 29, 77, 81;
Blood, 21, 27-3, 98;
    circulation 4, 15;
    sugar 20;
Blood Vessels, 52;
Blueberry, 38, 42;
Body, 5, 9, 38, 51, 52;
    adjusting 16, 67, 76, 105, 106;
    knowing your 2, 37;
    metabolism 12-15, 47-48;
Bones, 55;
    calcium 27;
Brain, 14, 16, 52, 98, 102;
Bread, 54, 80, 99, 100;
Breakfast, 1, 12, 17, 25, 37, 39, 66;
    bars 38;
Broccoli, 55, 62-63, 97;
Buffet, 49, 95;
BURGER KING, 9, 68, 70;
Butter, 26, 66, 100;
Calcium, 38, 98;
    foods with 27,
    sources of 53, 55;

Calorie, (s) 21, 22, 28, 29, 44-48, 53;
    count 2, 22, 65, 66, 67, 77, 93;
    low 9-15, 26, 39, 69-75, 79;
    alcohol 44;
    lunch 66;
    health risk 2;
    burning off 2, 9,
Cancer, 20, 38, 45, 98
Candy Bars, 25-27, 47
Canola oil, 61,
Capsaicin, 19,
Carrot, 7, 43, 59, 62, 63, 66;
Celery, 7, 40, 58, 59;
Clam, 58, 59;
Coconut, 104;
Collard Greens, 55;
Combo, 3, 20, 22;
Commitment, 76, 105;
Concentration, 37;
Cookie, (s) 26;
Cooking, 50, 51, 93;
Copper, 19, 26, 27;
Cranberries, 25, 40, 42;

Craving, (s) 45, 46, 66, 76, 82; 105-106;
   controlling 3, 7, 16, 1 8;
     food addiction 45, 46;
      snacking 25;

Cucumber, 40;

Cereal, 16, 17, 38, 54;

Diabetes, 21, 79, 8;
   causes 24, 44, 52;

Cheese, 9, 12, 38, 85, 95, 100, 103;
     food addiction 45, 65;
      low fat 46, 55;

Chicken, 10-12, 18, 50, 53, 56, 93-94 97, 65;

Children, obesity 24;

Diarrhea, 18, 27;

Diet, 2, 5;
     changing up 16, 51, 67;
     soda 24;
      exercise 29;

Digest, 10, 51, 56, 96;
     foods that helps with 15-19;
     red meat 51-52, 56;

Digestion, 15;
   water 17;

Digestive System, 18, 49, 82;

Dinner, (s) 1, 7, 48, 49, 79;
> frozen 93;
>> recipes 56-64;

Disease, 2, 20, 45;
> heart 20, 24, 98;
>> overeating 41;
>>> prevention 26, 38, 52, 102;
>>>> red meat 51;

Depression, 46, 77;

Desk, 4, 15, 28, 29, 30-36;

Doctors, 2, 78, 80, 81, 82;

Down Time, 5, 29;

Determination, 76;

Elevator, 4, 28-23;

Energy, 12-13, 28, 37, 78, 98;

Exercise, 1, 80;
> making time to 8, 29, 46;
>> home 77
>>> walking 28, 78,
>>>> pregnancy 81;

Experimenting, with new foods 7, 12,

Fast food, 1, 2, 3, 16, 20-25;
> places to eat 5, 9, 10, 11;

Fatty Acids, 26, 52, 101;

Fatty Foods, 16;
FDA, 82;
Fig, 26, 27;
Fish,
    baked 50, 52, 49, 56, 97, 99, 101-102;
      Catfish, 52;
        Trout 52;
          Tuna, 52;
Foliate, 27, 53;
Food addiction, 16, 45-47, 65;
Food Pyramid, 54, 55;
Fried, 54, 66, 96, 97, 99, 101-104;
Fries, 3, 11, 20-21, 45, 46, 50, 96;
Fruit, 49, 54, 80, 81, 83, 96-99, 109;
    losing weight 17,
      juice 24-27, 38-43, 44;
        food pyramid 54;
      organic 55;
Garlic, 98, 100;
Ginger Root, 38, 41-43;
GMO 93;
Granola Bar, 26, 38, 47, 83;
Grapefruit, 41;
Grease, 2, 10;
Grilling, 51-52;

Gym, 14, 29, 77;
Habits, 6, 12, 75, 80;
    breaking old 5, 29, 37, 46;
Hamburger, 3, 45;
    Burger King, 9,
Health, (y) 6, 7, 15, 16, 37, 47, 65;
    eating 3, 5, 9, 10, 11, 17, 25-27, 48-56;
      risk 2, 20-24;
Heart, 2;
    disease 20, 21, 24, 28-29, 38, 44, 98;
      attack 45;
High Fructose Corn Syrup, 16, 22- 24, 44, 55, 65;
Hormone, (s) 16;
Hunger, 5, 14, 39;
    snacking 76:
Ice cream, 46-47;
Indian, food 99;
Iron, 18, 20, 27, 56;
Italian, food 66, 100;
Japanese, food 101;
Juice, (r) 18, 24-25, 27, 38-39
Juicing, 38, 55;
Keyboard, 33-34;
KFC, 10;
Kiwi, 41;

Lamb, 60, 99;
Lasagna, 62;
Lemon,(ade) 22, 49, 57 60;
Lettuce 58, 65;
Lunch, 1-3, 15;
    digestion 16;
      music, 14;
        snacking before 25, 37, 76;
        menu 67-75;
Lifestyle, 37, 45, 82;
Lime, 41;
Magnesium, 19, 27, 53;
Mango, 41;
Mc Donald's, 11, 22, 68, 69, 71, 74;
Meal, 7, 11, 12, 23, 39, 41, 44, 48, 50, 65, 79-81, 93 96-104;
    low calorie 10,
Mediterranean, food
Melon, 38, 39;
Metabolism, 4-5, 12-15, 48-49;
    foods that help 17-19;
      exercise 28;
        taking the stairs 34;
      water 20;
Mexican, food 103;

Milk, 55, 53;
   low fat 24, 55;
     soy 40,55;
       coconut 104;
         almond 40;
           shakes 4;
Muscle, 13, 77, 78, 82;
   fat burning 15, 28-32;
Mushroom, 62, 84-85 94;
Mustard, 61;
Myth, 5;
Niacin, 56;
Nutrients, 19, 27, 38, 52, 53, 56, 78;
Nuts, 25, 26, 38, 52, 56, 65, 83, 98, 102;
Obesity, 2, 20, 98;
     children 24;
       red meat 52;
Oil, 50, 57, 59;
   fries 21;
    food pyramid 54;
Okra, 56;
Olive Oil, 100, 102;
Omega 3 fatty acids, 26, 52,   101-102;
Onions, 58-59, 62-63; 84-88;

Orange, 25;
    juice 41; 43, 61, 62;
Order, (ING) 3, 10-12, 22, 45;
    healthy 53, 65-66, 75, 79 95-99, 104;
Oven, 10, 53;
    baking 45, 50;
Parsley, 40, 57 60-61;
Pie, 46, 49;
Pineapple, 51;
Pizza, 53, 66, 84, 100;
Popcorn, 26
Potassium, 20, 27, 38, 53, 98;
Pounds,
    gaining, 42, 44, 49, 70;
    losing 27, 71;
Pretzels, 27;
Protein, 18, 20, 26, 28, 52-54, 56, 80, 98;
    bars 78-79;
Raspberry, 38, 40, 42;
Refrigerator, 47;
Relax, 8;
    music 14;
      roasted 10;
        exercise 36;

Results, 4, 29, 76;
Riboflavin, 56;
Rice, 50, 62;
Pedometer, 28;
Pepper, 57-65, 84-90, 104;
    chili 19;
Phosphorus, 19, 26;
Saccharin, 45;
Salad, 1, 9, 22, 57, 65 100,102, 104;
Salmon, 52, 57 89, 101, 102;
Salt, 21, 26, 27, 45, 56-63, 65, 83, 86-88;
    kosher 89;
Seafood, 56, 99, 102, 104;
Seasoned, 50, 51;
Shies-kabobs, 51;
Smoothies, 17, 39-43, 66;
Soda, 22- 24, 49, 65;
Sodium, 21, 26, 27, 53;
Soft drink, 22-23, 44, 81;
    value 3;
Spinach, 40, 55, 63-65, 98, 100;
Starving, myth 5;
    yourself 13, 49;
Steam, (ed) 49;
Stew, (ing), 50, 99;

Stomach,
>   metabolism 13-18;

Strawberry, 38;
>   milkshake 4;

Substance Abuse, 44;
Subway, 10, 69, 73;
Success, 5, 6, 14, 45, 52, 106;
Sucralose, 45;
Sugar, 5, 16-17, 20, 45, 54;
>   brown 61,
>   pure 22;
>   soda 44;
>   smoothies 39;

Sweeteners, 45;
Taco Bell, 12, 72, 74;
Thai, food 104;
Thermogenesis, 19;
Tomato, 65, 98, 100;
Treadmill, 28, 77;
Variety, 7, 10, 26, 48;
>   at dinner 56, 80, 93, 95, 99;
>   exercise 77;

Vegetable, 56;
Vegetarian, 66;
Vending Machine, 1, 25;

Vinaigrette, 65;
Vitamin, A 19;
    B 19, 20; 26, 27;
      B-6 19, 27, 53;
        B-12 98;
          C 19;
            D 18, 52;
              E 26;
Walking, 5;
    exercise 29, 78, 81;
    taking the stairs 4, 28,
Water, 3, 5, 14, 22 44-46, 55, 106;
    digestion 17;
      hydration 20;
        flavored 25, 45, 81;
Watermelon, 43,
Weight loss, 1, 22, 24, 47, 105;
    alcohol 44;
      digestion 15;
        healthy 19-21, 37, 48;
          unhealthy weight loss 13;
            pill 82;
              programs 78-81;
            surgery 82;
Wendy's, 3, 10, 68, 71,72, 74;

Whole Grains, 16, 19, 26, 27, 38, 54, 56, 83, 100, 102;
Willpower, 46;
Work, (ing) 1, 5, 14, 17-19, 48, 66;
    snacking 25, 83;
      staying active 4, 8, 15, 28-36;
Yoga, 81;
    office 30;
Yogurt, 11, 27, 38, 41, 47, 68
    Greek 98
Zinc, 20, 27, 56;

About the Author

V.L. Jenkins is a former fast food worker who has owned his own auto repair business, sold rental properties and also was a cross country driver visiting over forty states throughout America. A hard worker and determined entrepreneur who after a few minor setbacks from recent global economic strife decided to take up his craft of writing full time.

Having studied at numerous writing workshops throughout the state, he also has extensive studies in health and nutrition.

In his spare time he writes various novels and is a creative artist and musician as well. He currently lives in Detroit, MI.

To contact please send testimonials, confessions or suggestions to therealunlimiteduniverse1@gmail.com and receive info on upcoming releases from V.L. Jenkins or Universal Unlimited Publishing.

Made in the USA
Columbia, SC
09 March 2021